Fanny's guide to Flirting

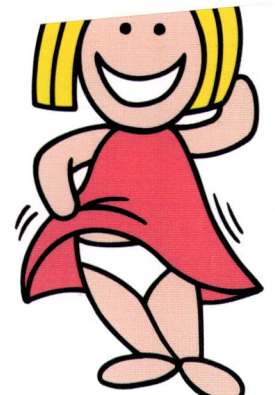

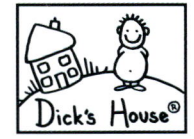

Dick's House®

First published 2002 by Contender Books
Contender Books is a division of
The Contender Entertainment Group
48 Margaret Street
London W1W 8SE

1 3 5 7 9 10 8 6 4 2

Fanny's Guide to Flirting © 2002 Pineapple Enterprises Limited
All rights reserved.
Dick's House® is a registered trademark of Pineapple Enterprises Limited

By Susie Jarman
Illustrations by Keiron Ward

No part of this publication may be reproduced, stored in a retrieval system, or transmitted in any form, or by any means, electrical, mechanical, photocopying, recording or otherwise without the prior permission of the publisher or a licence permitting restricted copying

ISBN 1-84357-001-7

Printed in Italy

Also published by Contender Books: DICK'S GUIDE TO GETTING IT

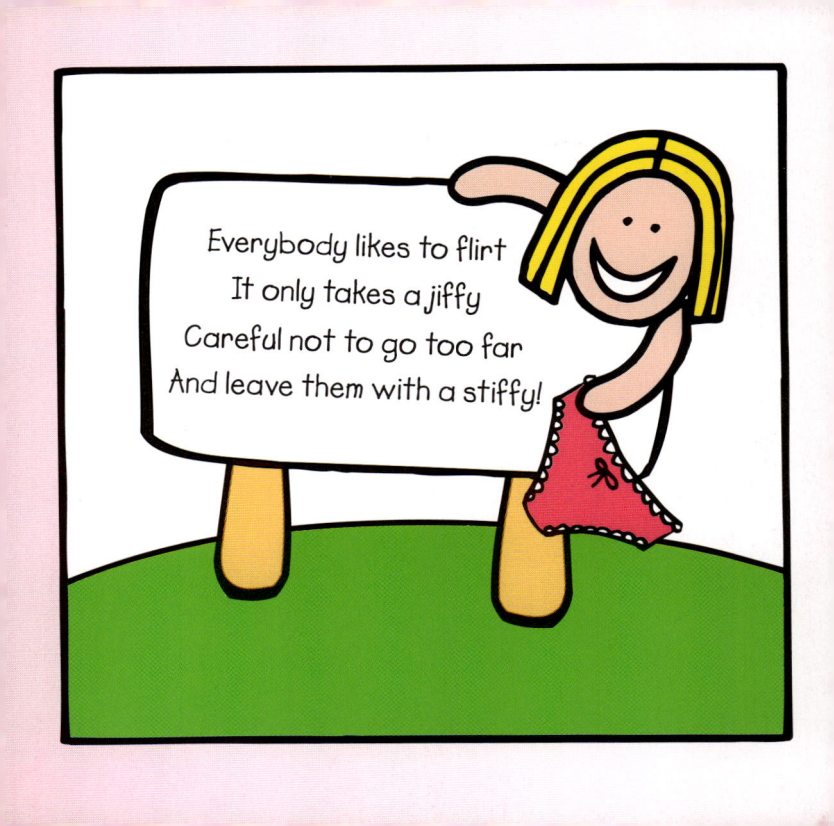

Everybody likes to flirt
It only takes a jiffy
Careful not to go too far
And leave them with a stiffy!

Flirting is great fun and what's more it's good for us!

Men are easy to flirt with as they have big egos and their brains are in their pants...

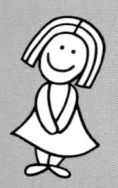

The male brain

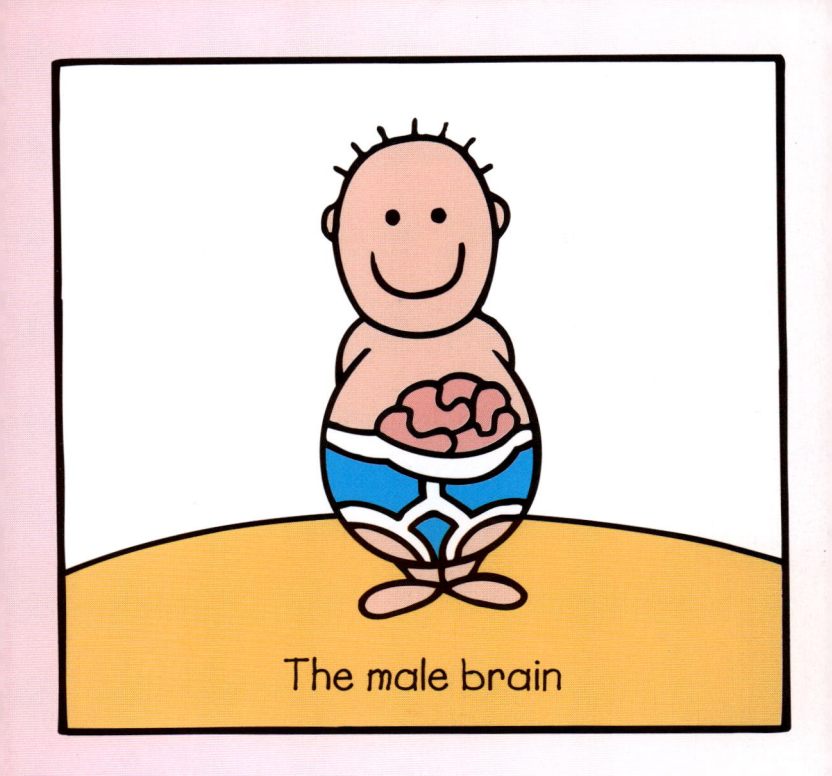

What is flirting?

Flirting can be as subtle as a smile!

Gestures, body language and chit chat are all part of the game...

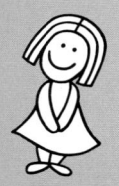

"Does my bum look big in this?"

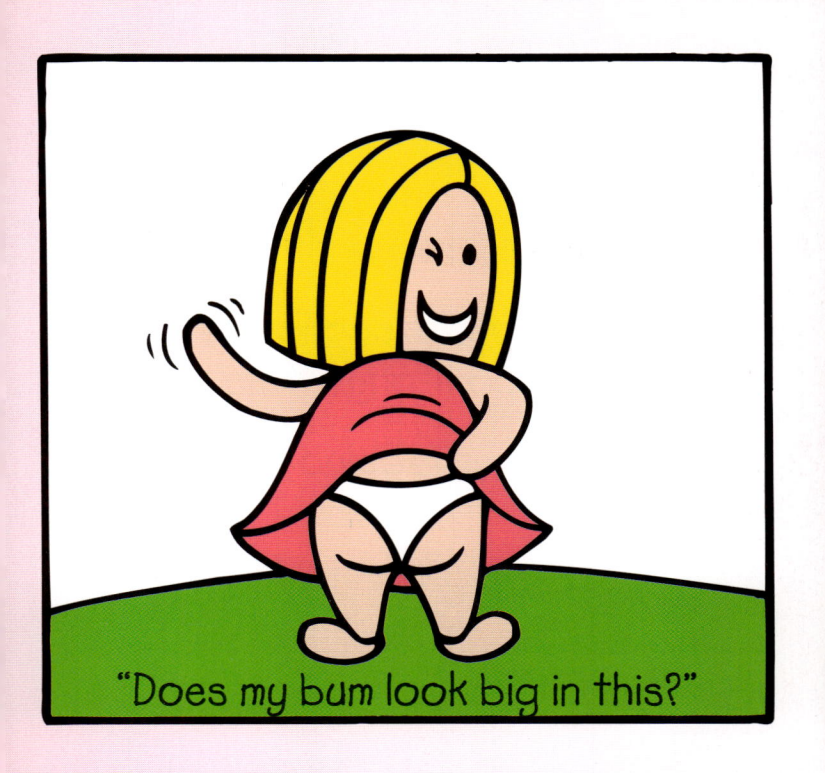

Places to flirt

An experienced flirter
can do it anywhere!

Use your imagination...

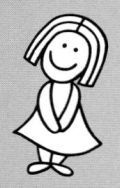

FRUIT + VAG

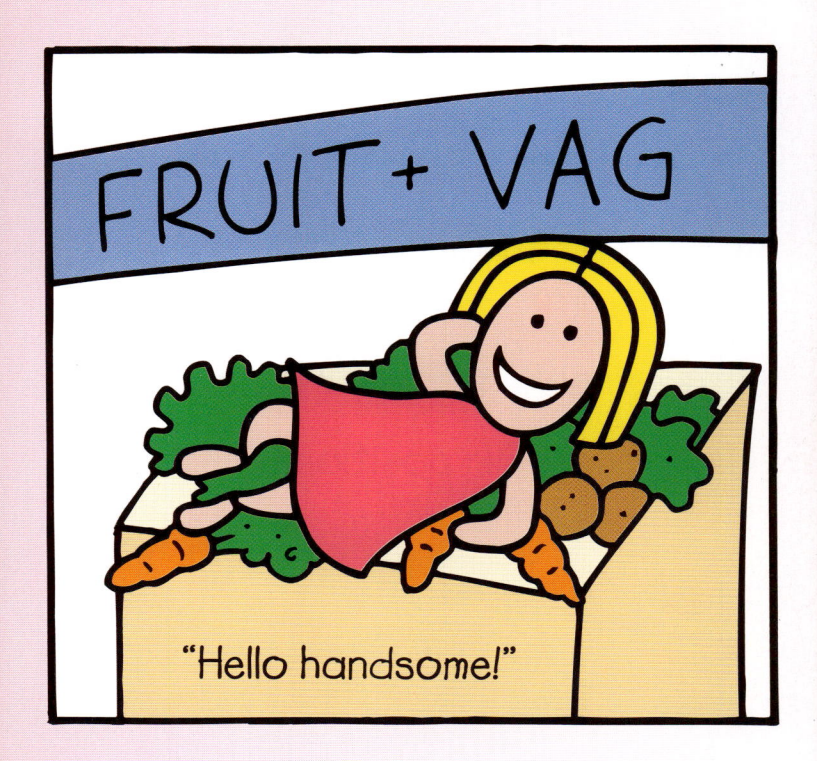

"Hello handsome!"

Power flirting

Don't forget to flirt at work -
it helps us get what we want...

Put yourself in position for a rise!

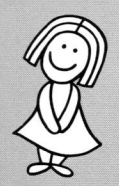

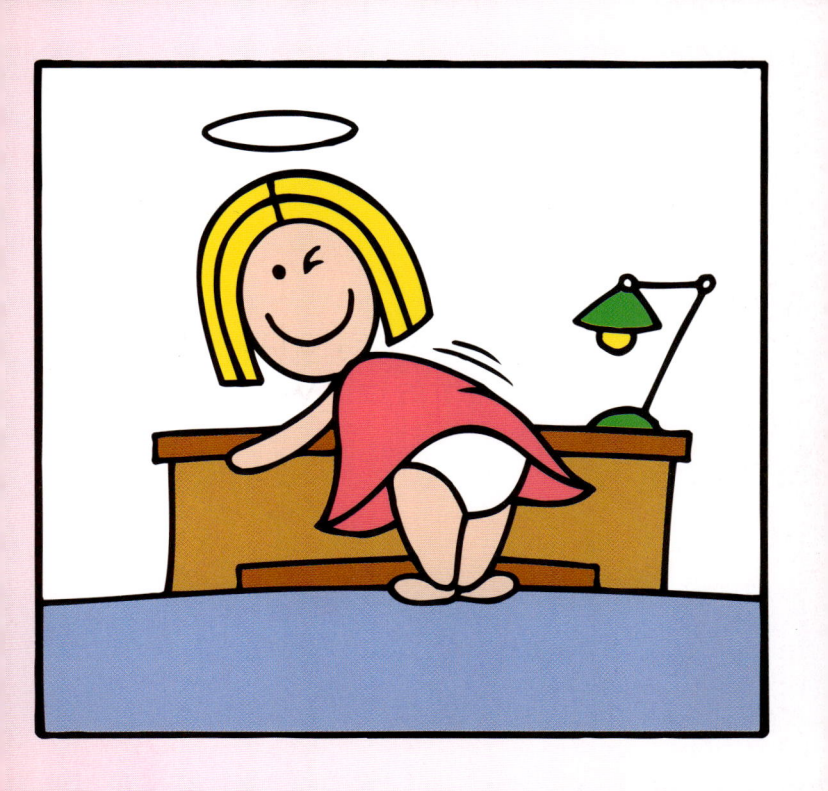

No go areas

He may be drop-dead gorgeous,
but there's always a time and place...

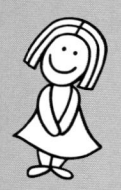

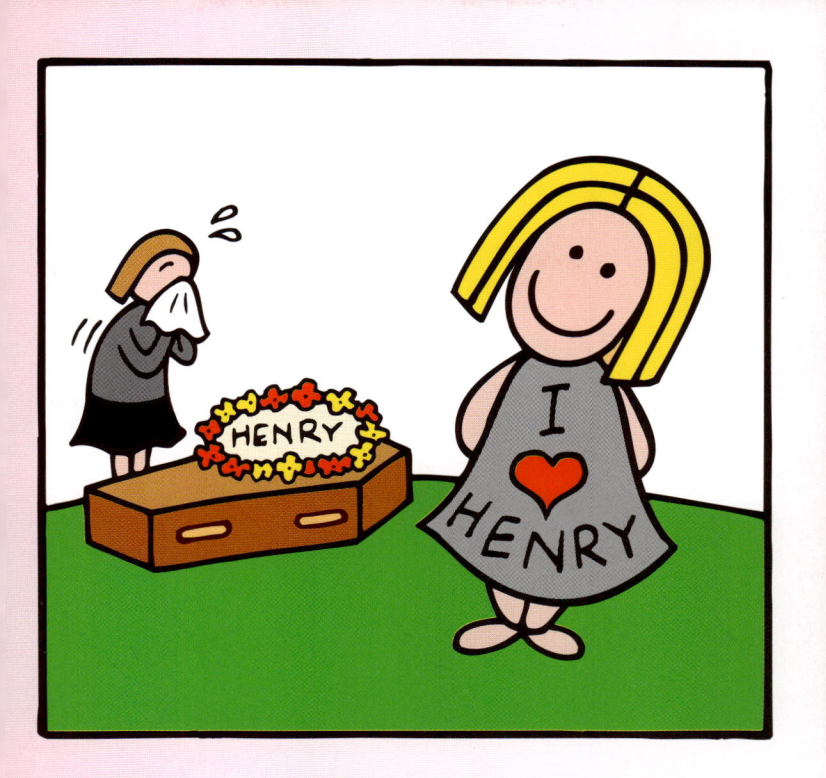

Prepare to flirt

Make an effort!

Men like women who look and smell sexy...

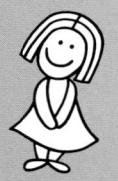

Fanny keeps her pussy clean

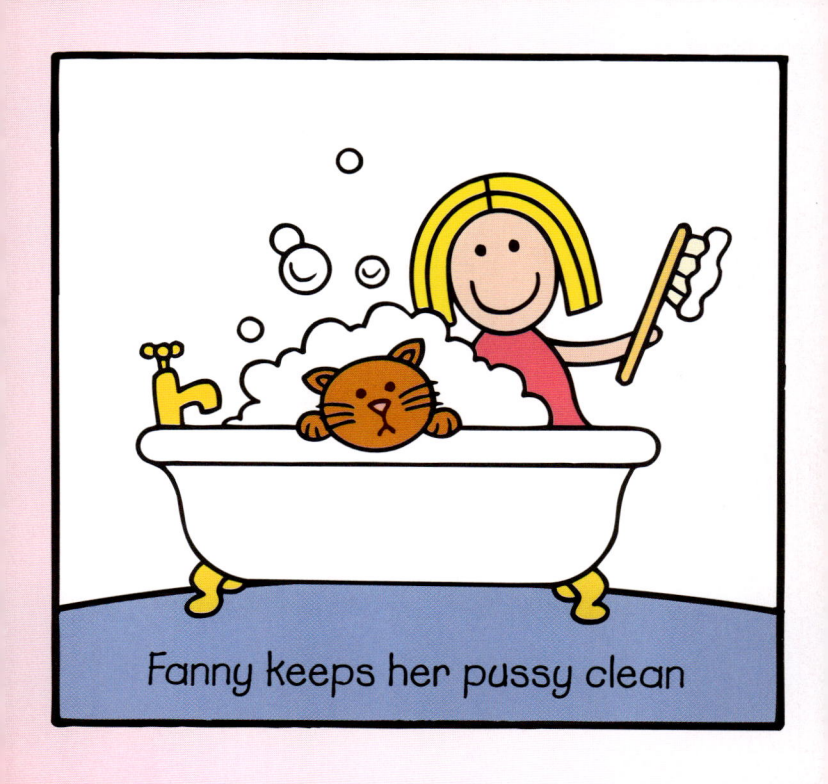

Make your entrance

Be sure to get noticed,
but be cool...

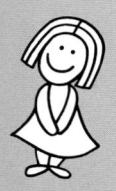

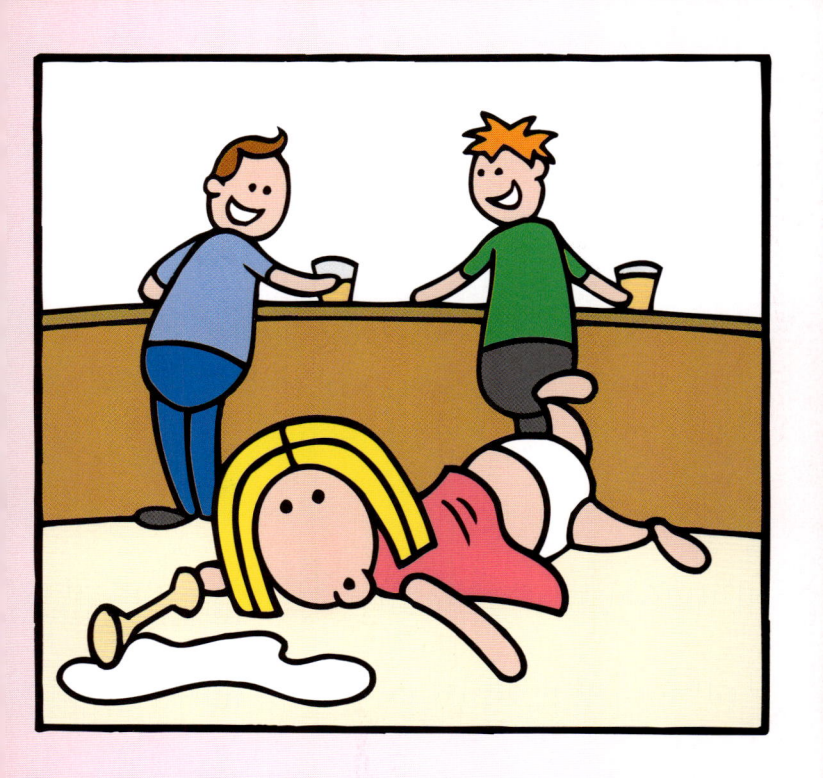

Choose your victim

Okay, so most men are easy,
but some are easier
than others...

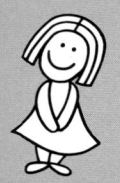

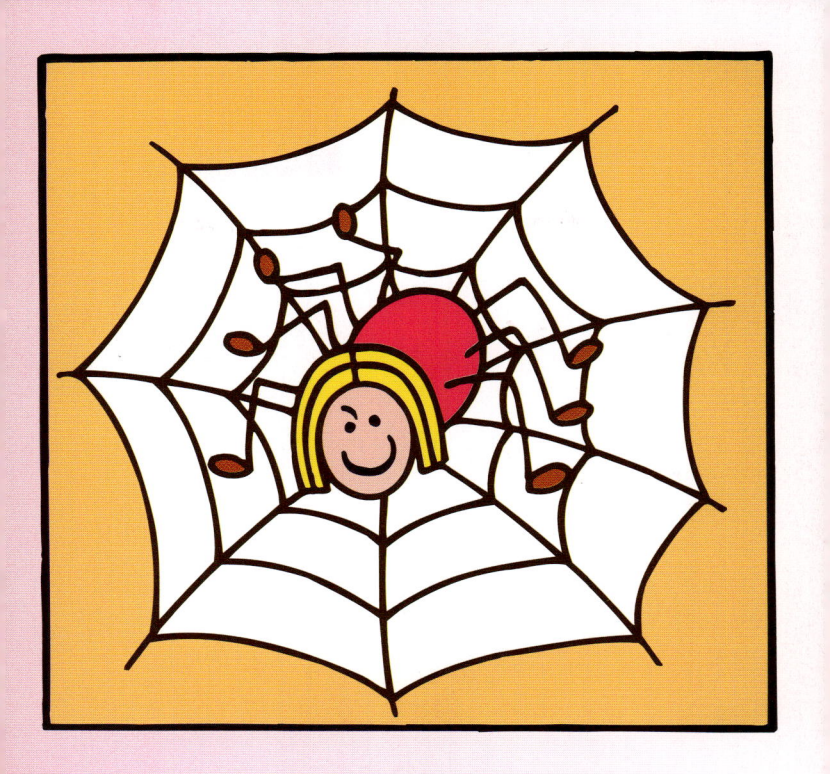

Dead Certs

Young men

Very keen and easy to manipulate...

May come in their pants!

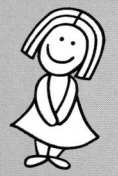

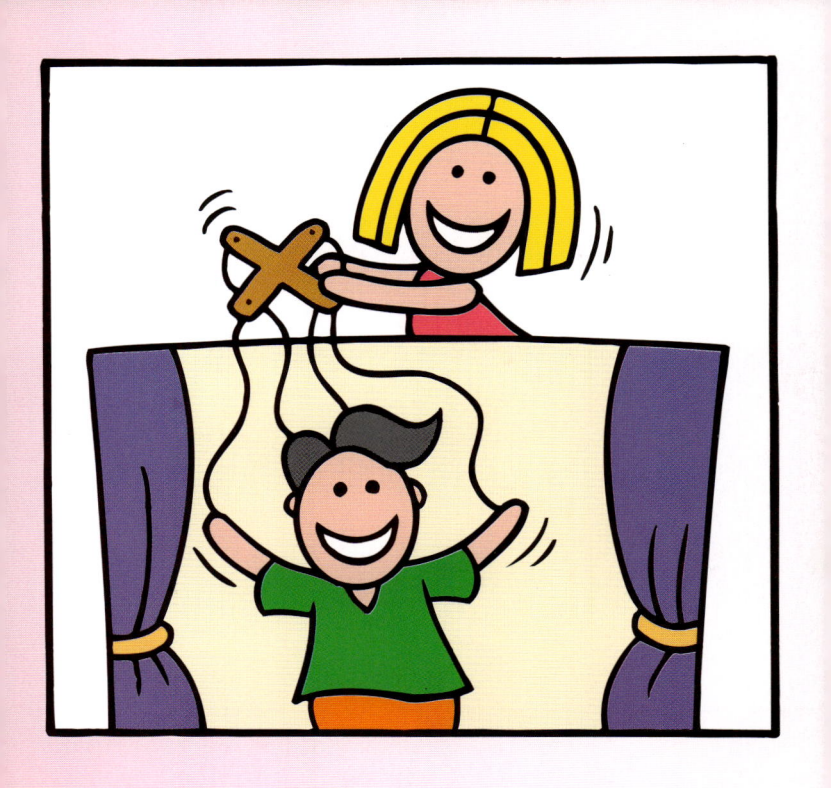

Middle-aged men

Easy to flatter and love female company.

Probably married and not getting it!

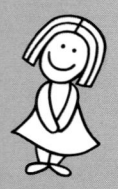

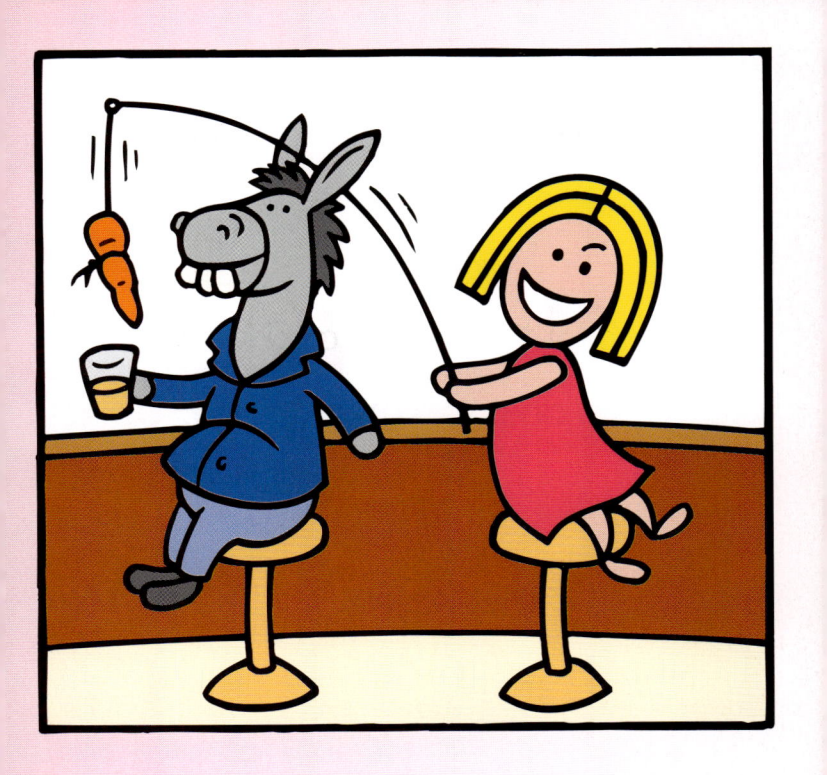

Gym junkies

Think they look good.

Big willies are not their strong point!

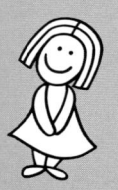

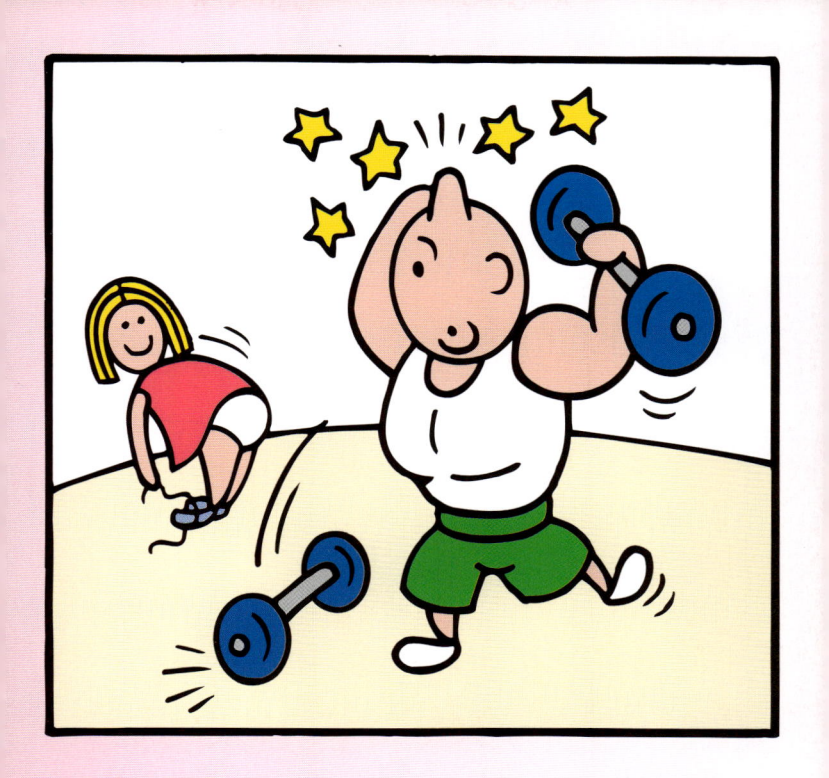

Business men

Usually think they're in with a chance...

Like to use their flexible friend
and charge it to expenses!

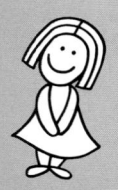

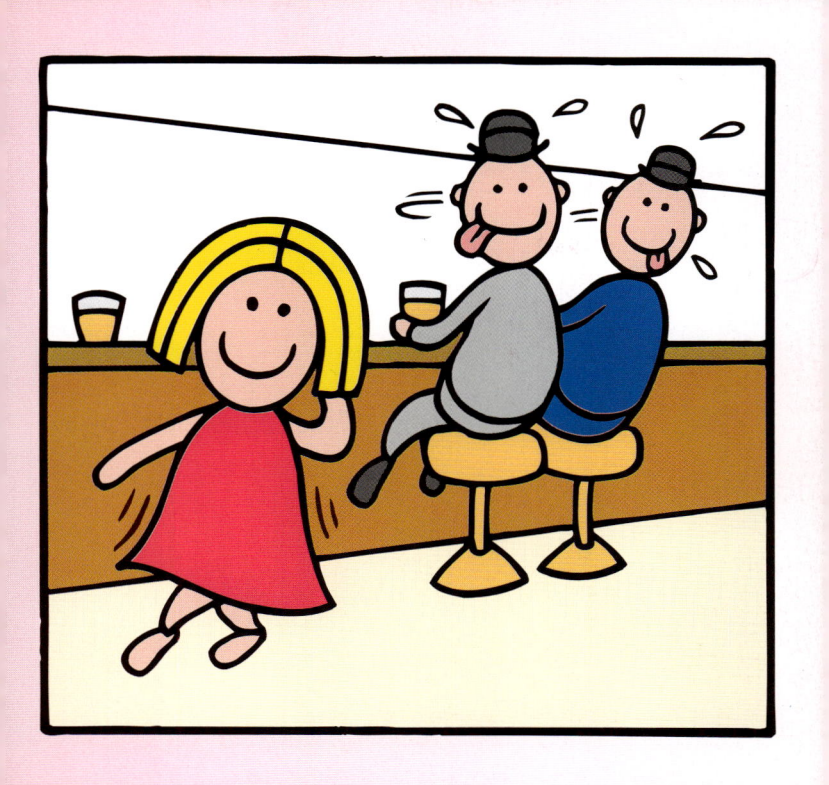

Unpredictable types

Mummies boys

Could be too scared and may cry...

Only used to keeping mummy happy!

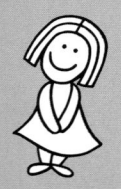

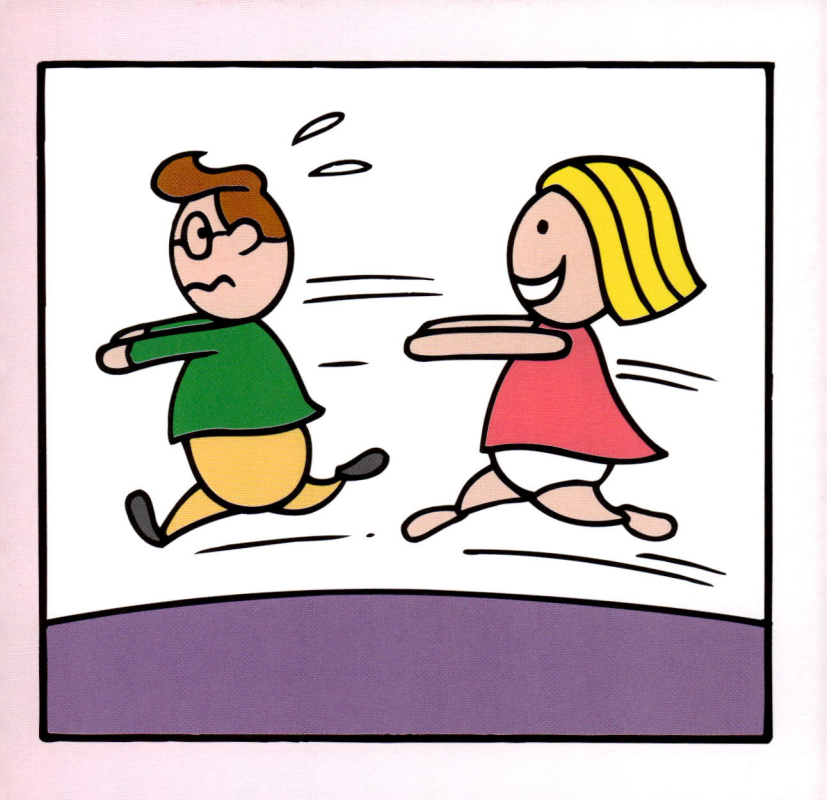

Ugly men

May think you're taking the piss,
but are grateful anyway.

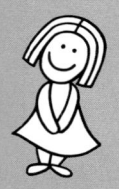

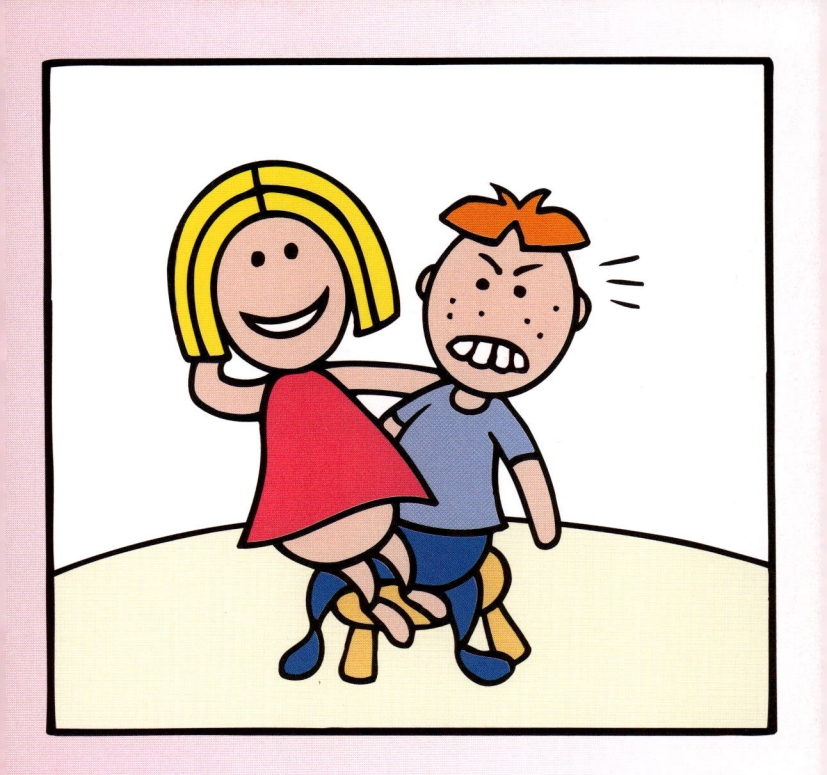

Couch potatoes

Usually too lazy to flirt back...

Convince him he's watching the wrong box!

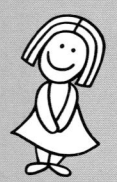

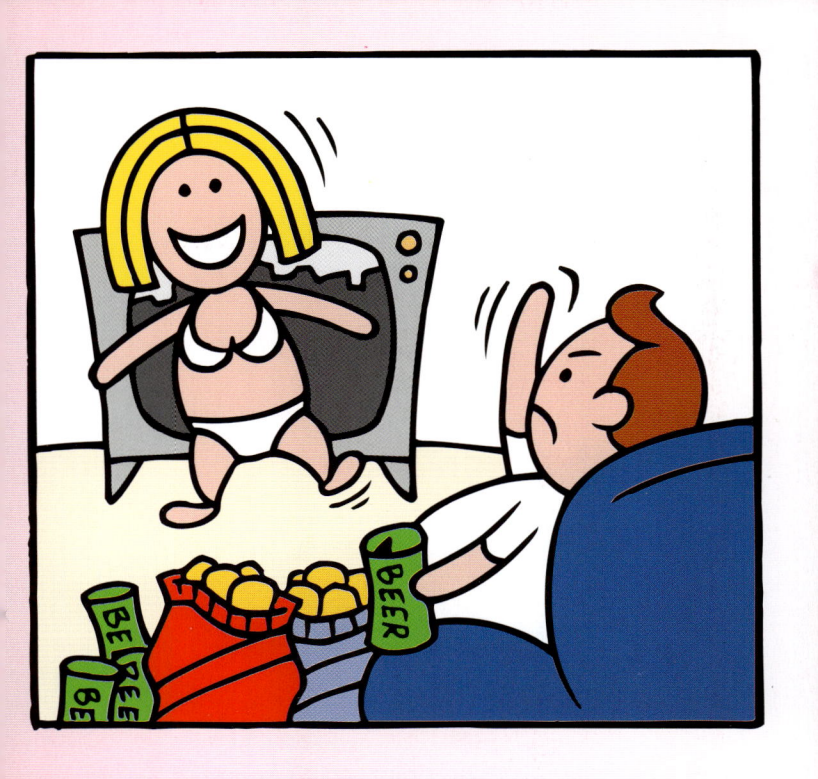

Men of the cloth

A difficult one as they tend to abstain.

Those that don't, usually prefer men.

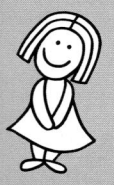

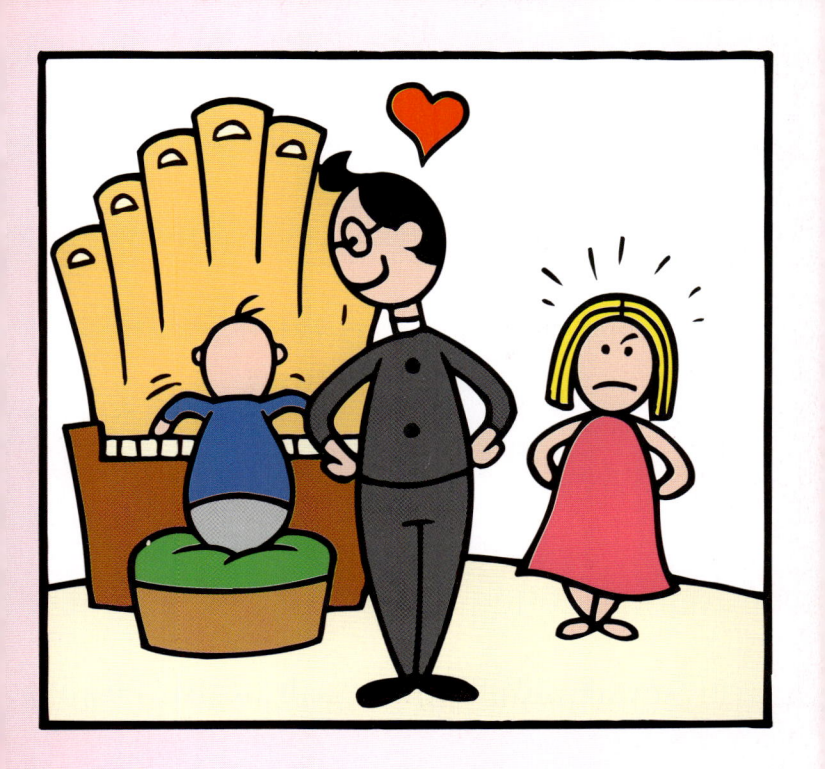

Beware

Appearances can be deceptive...

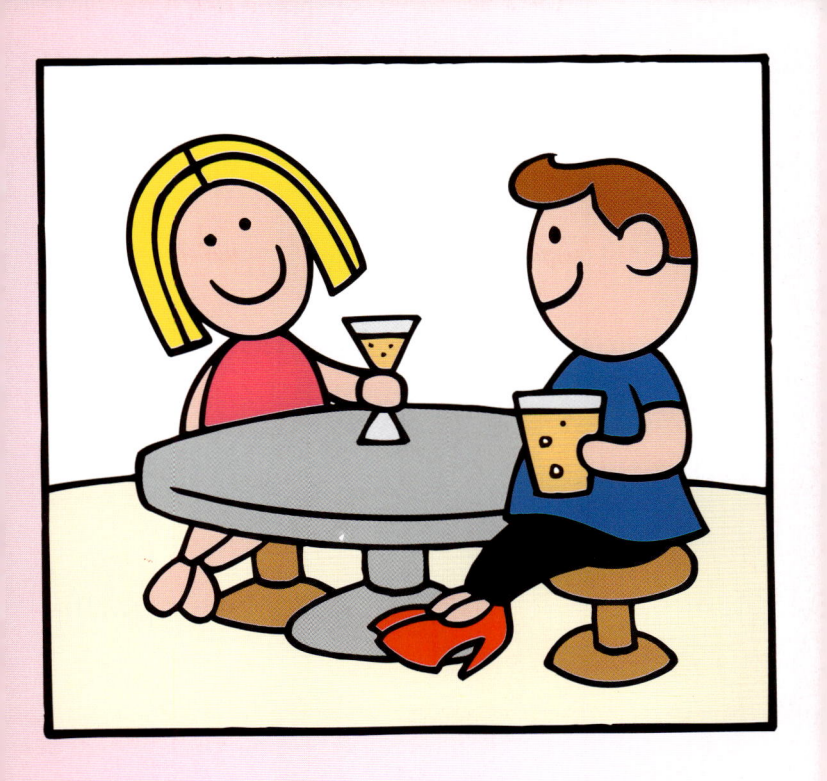

Test the water

Try flirting a little
to gauge the reaction...

"Excuse me, have you got a stiffy?"

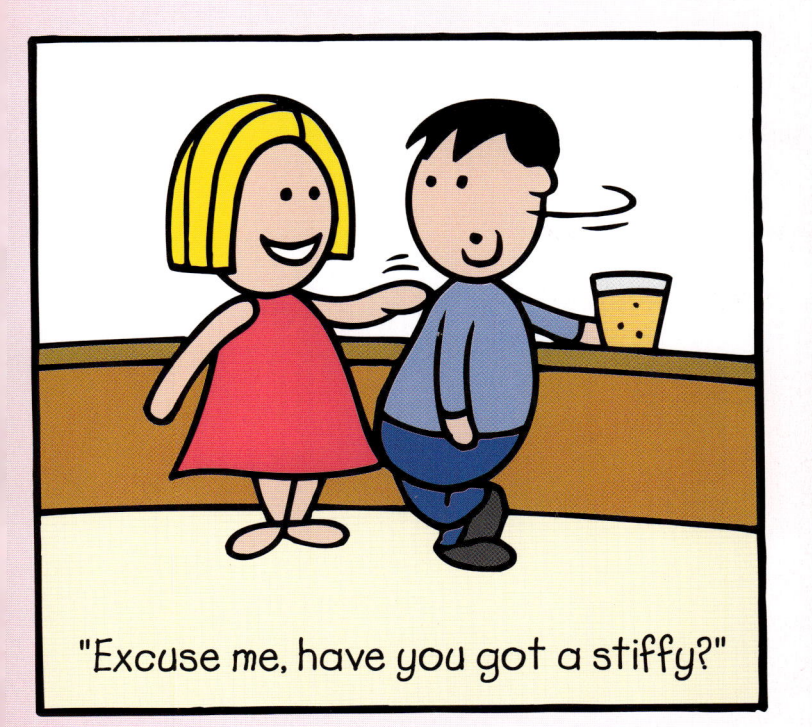

Always check out their credentials...

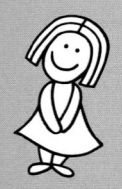

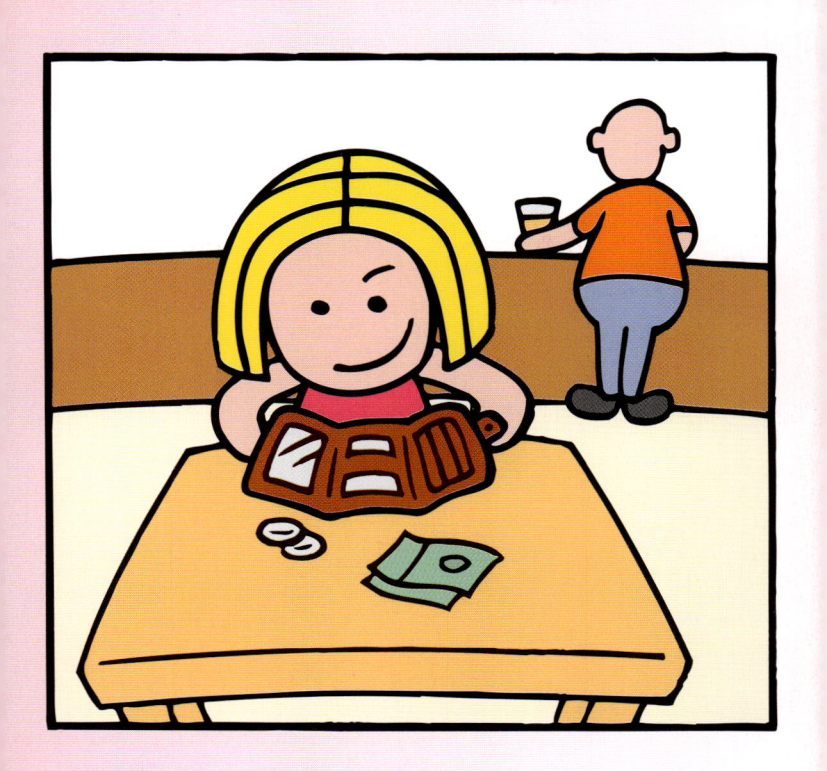

Top tips

Men like talking about themselves...

Don't yawn or they'll think you're ready for bed!

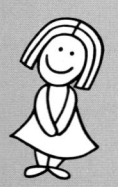

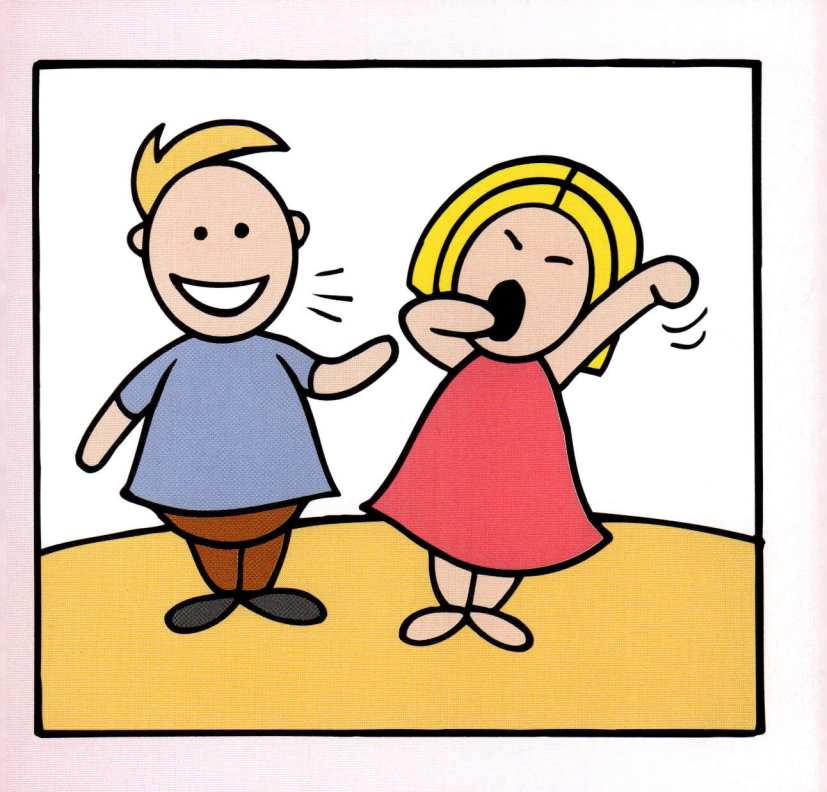

Don't be obvious...

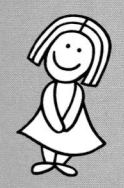

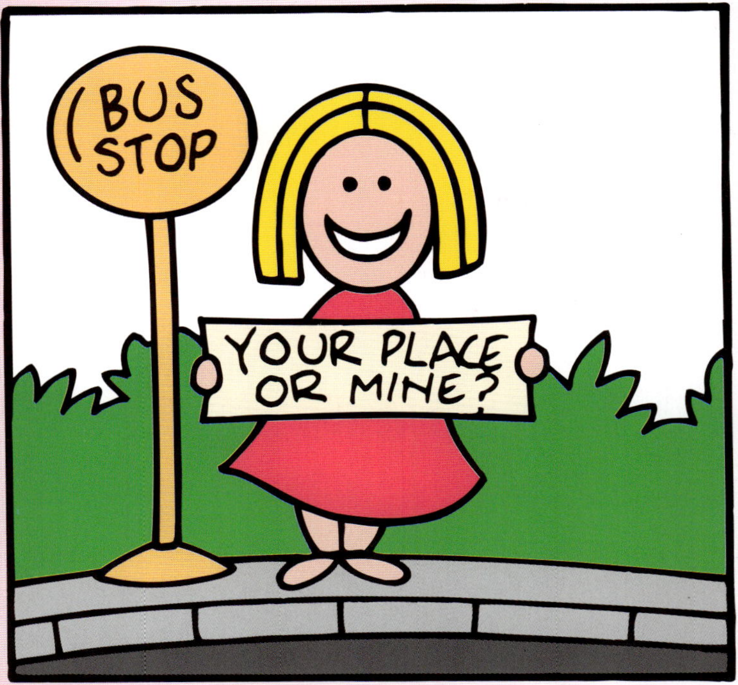
BUS STOP
YOUR PLACE OR MINE?

Don't overdo the body language...

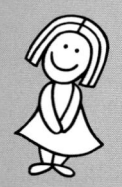

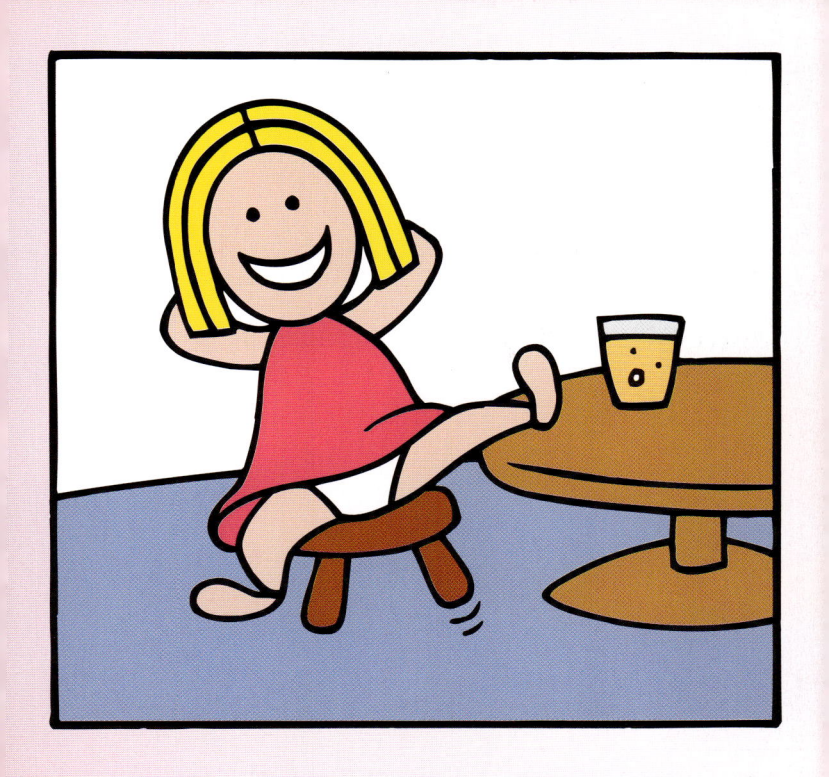

Don't act too desperate...

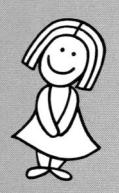

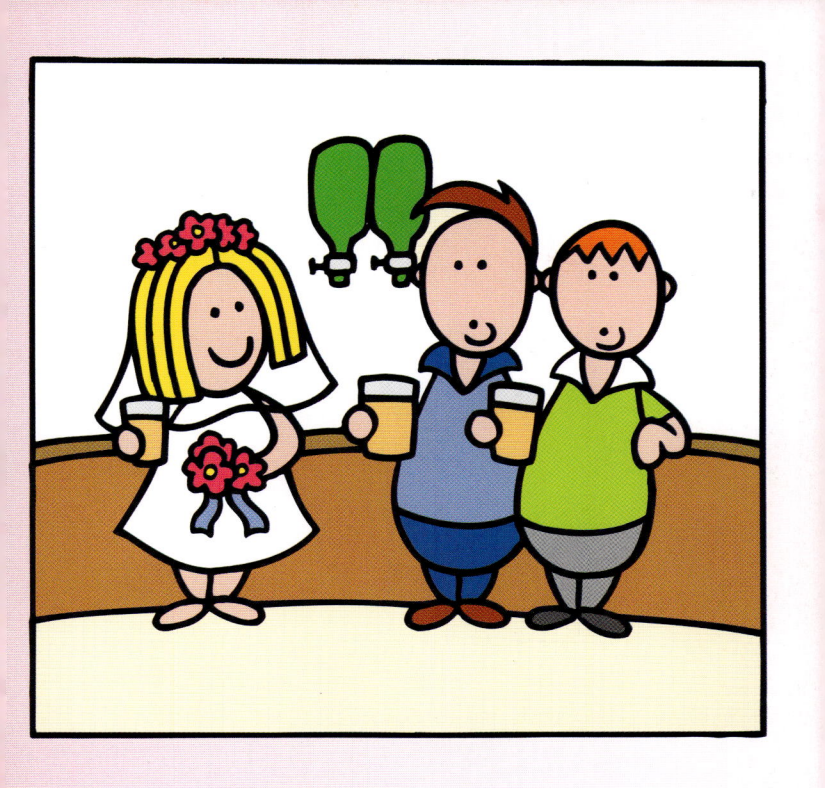

Remember, you're the one pushing the buttons...

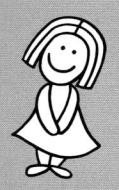

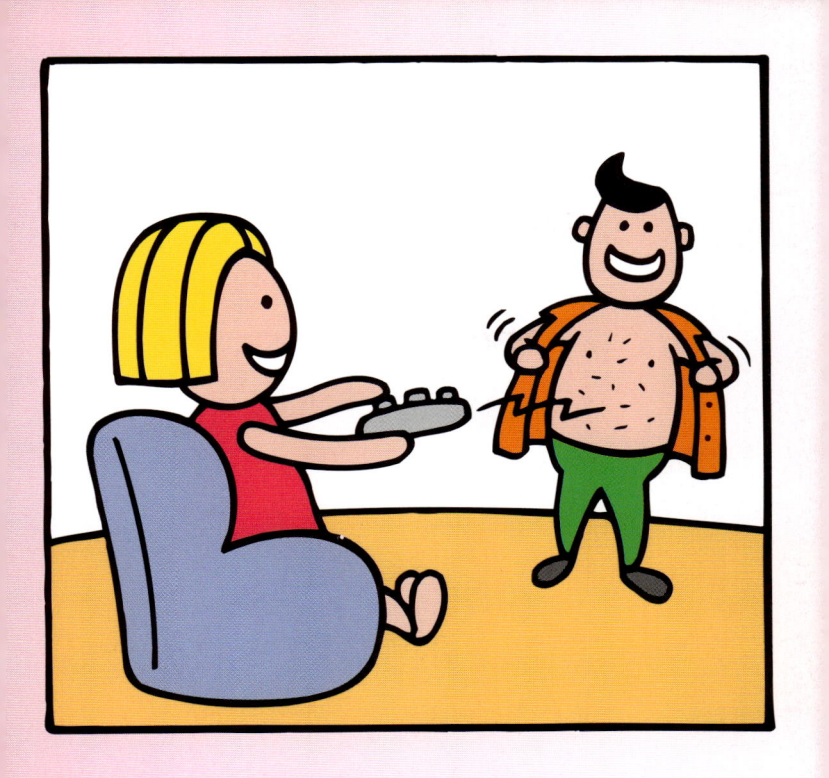

Use your intuition

Know when it's not working...

You've had his brother anyway!

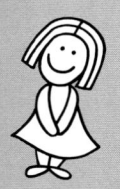

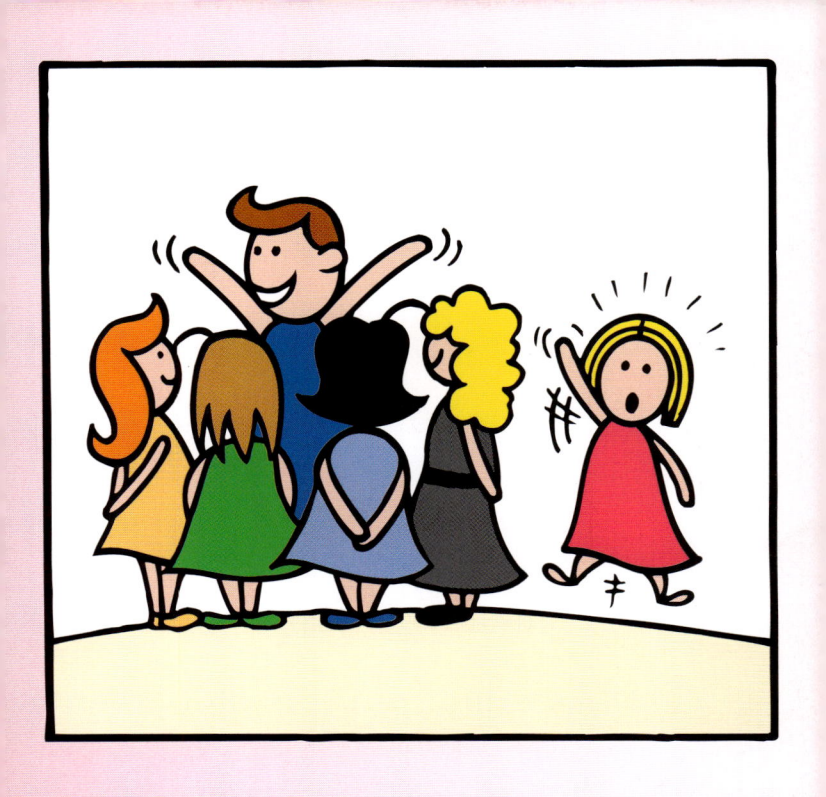

And move on to Plan B...

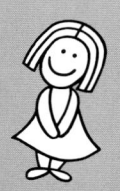

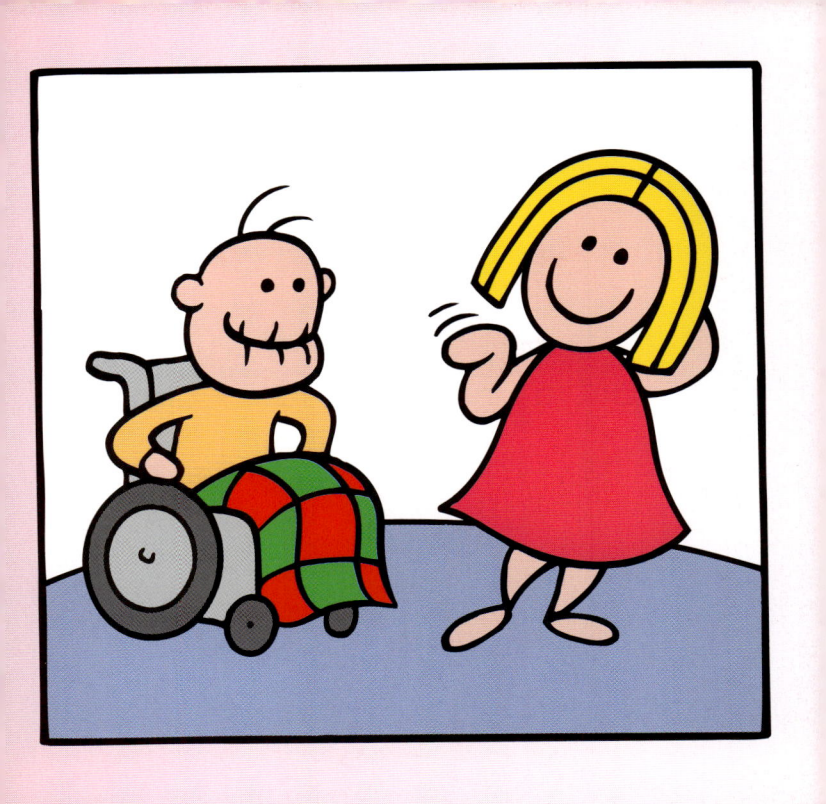

Go in for the kill

He may be incontinent,
but at least he's loaded!

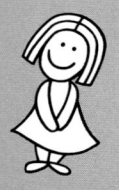

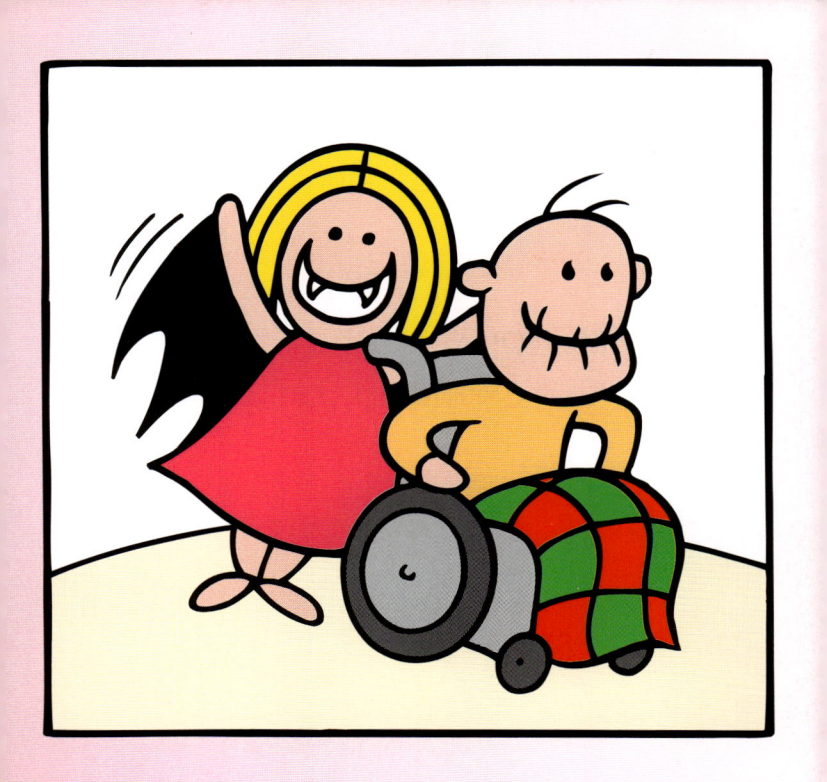

Be careful

You may get more than you bargained for...

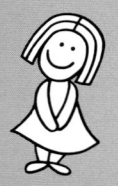

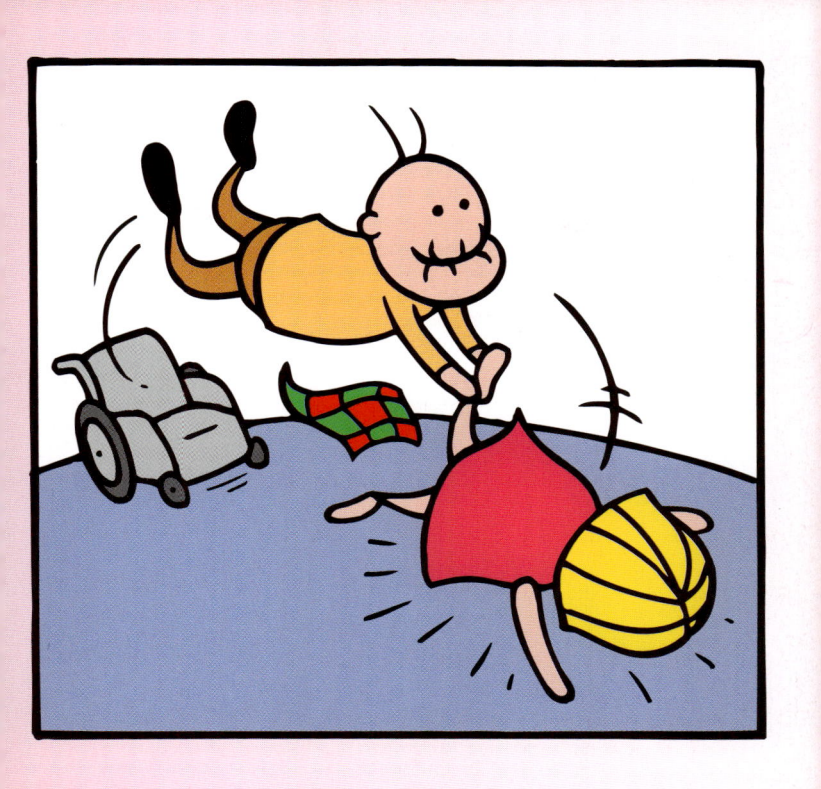

Know your escape route

If all else fails,
make a quick exit...

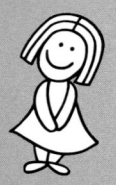

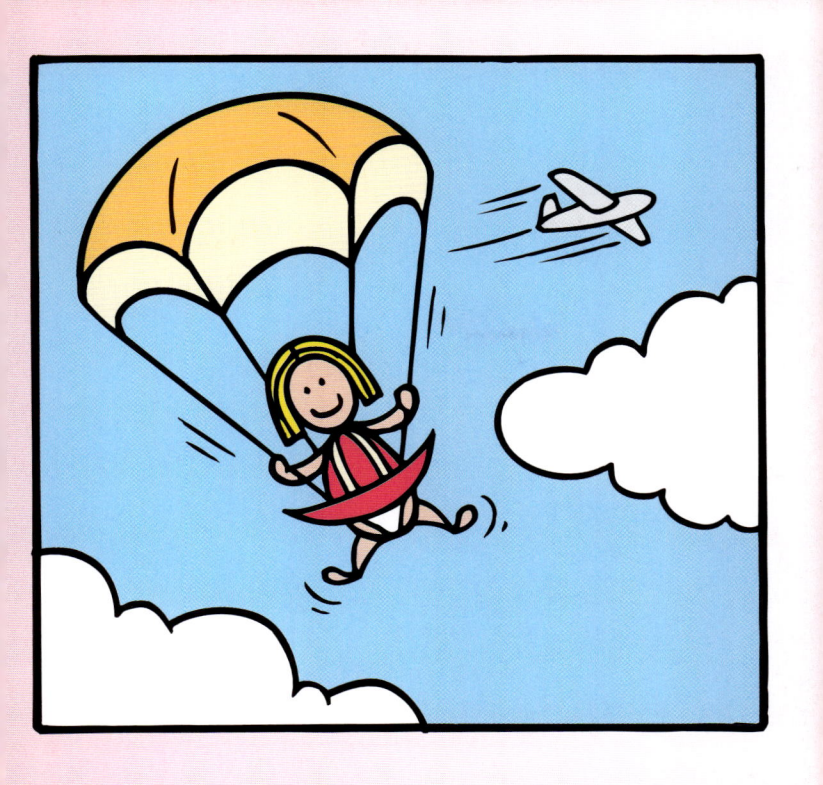

The end

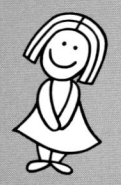

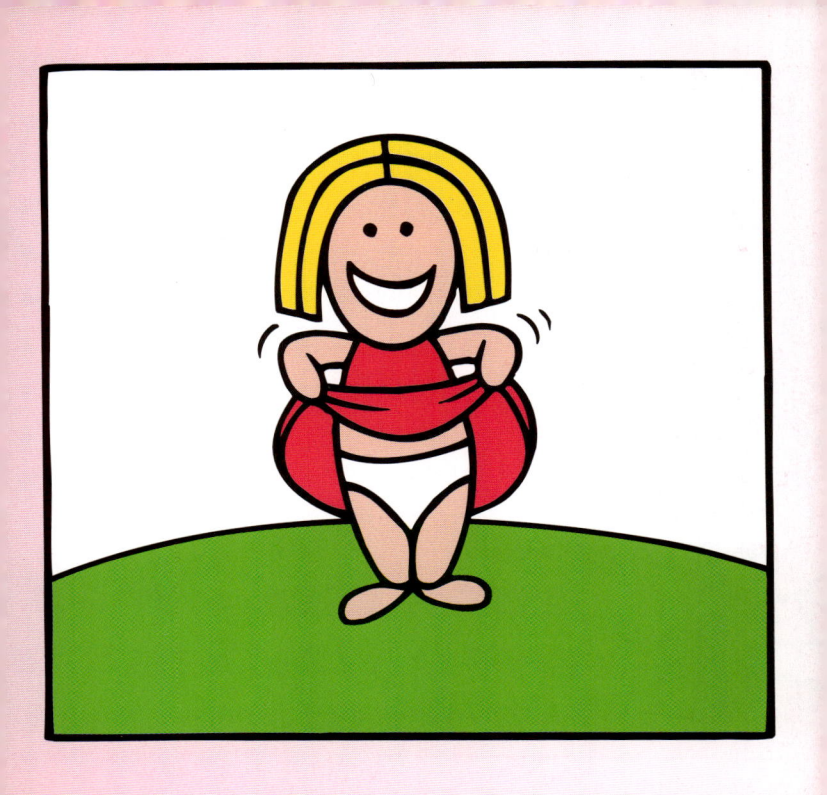

Get your Dick's House mobile goodies
Call 0906 553 4028*

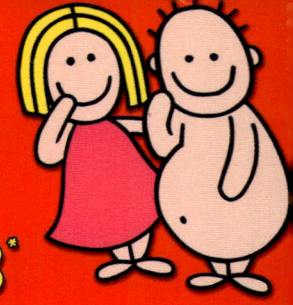

Calls cost £1/minute from a landline. Calls from mobiles may be more than £1 per minute.

Press 1 to send a flirty anonymous text message.
Press 2 to play a prank and listen to your friend being fooled!

*Call duration and cost depend on how long you stay on-line to select an anonymous text or prank call.

Get your Dick's House logo. Text FANNY followed by the name of your chosen logo to 8700
e.g. FANNY CHICK

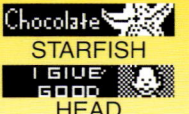

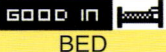

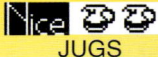

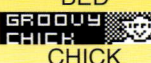

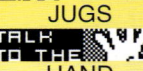

| Chocolate STARFISH | GOOD IN BED | Nice JUGS |
| I GIVE GOOD HEAD | GROOVY CHICK | TALK TO THE HAND |

Cost per logo: approximately £3.12. Vodafone, Cellnet/O2 and Orange subscribers only. You may receive further offers/info. To unsubscribe please text INFO STOP to 8700.

For Customer Care please call 0870 906 3434 (National Rate). Users must be 18 years +. Promoters: iTouch UK Ltd, 57-63 Scrutton Street, London EC2A 4PF. For more Dick's House mobile goodies go to www.itouch.co.uk/dicks

POWERED BY iTOUCH MOBILE